DAILY FITNESS MOTIVATION

365 DAYS OF THE BEST MOTIVATIONAL QUOTES FOR EXERCISE, WEIGHTLOSS, SELF-DISCIPLINE, TRAINING, BODYBUILDING, DIETING AND LIVING A HEALTHY LIFESTYLE.

Mick Kremling

"MAN CANNOT REMAKE HIMSELF WITHOUT SUFFERING, FOR HE IS BOTH THE MARBLE AND THE SCULPTOR."

DAY 2

"A YEAR FROM NOW, YOU'RE GOING TO WISH YOU STARTED TODAY."

"DO NOT PRAY FOR
AN EASY LIFE,
PRAY FOR THE
STRENGTH TO
ENDURE A
DIFFICULT ONE."

-BRUCE LEE

DAY 4

"PAIN IS WEAKNESS LEAVING THE BODY"

"COURAGE IS NOT HAVING THE STRENGTH TO GO ON. IT IS GOING ON WHEN YOU DON'T HAVE THE STRENGTH."

DAY 6

"INDECISION AND DELAY ARE THE PARENTS OF FAILURE."

-GEORGE CANNING

DAY 7

"YOUR FUTURE IS DETERMINED BY WHAT YOU DO TODAY, NOT TOMORROW."

"WHEN YOU FEEL LIKE QUITTING. THINK ABOUT WHY YOU STARTED."

"A FIT, HEALTHY BODY, THAT IS THE BEST FASHION STATEMENT."

-JESS C. SCOTT

DAY 10

"ACCOMPLISHMENT WILL PROVE TO BE A JOURNEY, NOT A DESTINATION."

-DWIGHT D. EISENHOWER

"THERE'S A DIFFERENCE BETWEEN KNOWING THE PATH AND WALKING THE PATH."

"THE ACT OF GETTING STRONG DOESN'T START IN THE GYM, IT STARTS IN YOUR HEAD"

-LISBETH DARSH

"TO KEEP THE BODY IN GOOD HEALTH IS A DUTY... OTHERWISE WE SHALL NOT BE ABLE TO KEEP OUR MIND STRONG AND CLEAR."

-Buddha

DAY 14

"YOU DIDN'T COME THIS FAR TO ONLY COME THIS FAR."

"THE LION DOES NOT CONCERN ITSELF WITH THE OPINIONS OF THE SHEEP."

DAY 16

"WHEN YOU'VE GOT SOMETHING TO PROVE, THERE'S NOTHING BETTER THAN A CHALLENGE."

-TERRY BRADSHAW

DAY 17

"DON'T STOP WHEN IT HURTS, STOP WHEN IT'S DONE."

DAY 18

"THIS IS YOUR WORLD. SHAPE IT OR SOMEONE ELSE WILL."

" I AM INDEED A KING, BECAUSE I KNOW HOW TO RULE MYSELF." -

Pietro Aretino

DAY 20

"DIE WITH MEMORIES, NOT DREAMS."

DAY 21

"IF IT IS IMPORTANT TO YOU, THEN YOU WILL FIND A WAY. IF IT IS NOT THEN YOU WILL FIND AN EXCUSE."

"EVERY BATTLE IS WON BEFORE IT IS FOUGHT."

-SUN TZU

"YOU HAVE TO PUSH PAST YOUR PERCEIVED LIMITS, PUSH PAST THAT POINT YOU THOUGHT WAS AS FAR AS YOU CAN GO."

-DREW BREES

"THERE IS A BEAST WITHIN EVERYONE, THAT STIRS WHEN YOU PUT A BARBELL IN THEIR HANDS."

DAY 25

"YOU DON'T DROWN BY FALLING IN WATER, YOU DROWN BY STAYING THERE."

"ASK NOT FOR A LIGHTER BURDEN, BUT FOR BROADER SHOULDERS."

"IF YOU WANT SOMETHING YOU'VE NEVER HAD, THEN YOU MUST DO SOMETHING YOU'VE NEVER DONE."

"THE MAN WHO MOVES A MOUNTAIN BEGINS BY CARRYING AWAY SMALL STONES."

DAY 29

"TRAIN LIKE A BEAST, LOOK LIKE A BEAUTY."

FATE WHISPERED TO THE WARRIOR "YOU CANNOT DEFEAT THE STORM" THE WARRIOR WHISPERED BACK "I AM THE STORM"

DAY 31

"ONE WORKOUT AT A TIME. ONE DAY AT A TIME. ONE WEEK AT A TIME."

DAY 32

"A CONSTANT STRUGGLE, A CEASELESS BATTLE TO BRING SUCCESS FROM INHOSPITABLE SURROUNDINGS, IS THE PRICE FOR ALL GREAT ACHIEVEMENTS."

-Orison Swett Marden

DAY 33

"VICTORY IS RESERVED FOR THOSE WILLING TO PAY ITS PRICE."

-SUN TZU

"ONE OF THE GREATEST MOMENTS IN LIFE, REALIZING THAT TWO WEEKS AGO YOUR BODY COULDN'T DO WHAT IT JUST DID."

"PHYSICAL FITNESS IS NOT ONLY ONE OF THE MOST IMPORTANT KEYS TO A HEALTHY BODY, IT IS THE BASIS OF DYNAMIC AND CREATIVE INTELLECTUAL ACTIVITY."

– JOHN F. KENNEDY

DAY 36

"DECIDE. COMMIT. SUCCEED."

"IF A MAN ACHIEVES VICTORY OVER THIS BODY, WHO IN THE WORLD CAN EXERCISE POWER OVER HIM? HE WHO RULES HIMSELF RULES OVER THE WHOLE WORLD."

–VINOBA BHAVE

"WHEN IT COMES TO EATING RIGHT AND EXERCISING, THERE IS NO 'I'LL START TOMORROW.' TOMORROW IS DISEASE."

-V.L. ALLINEAR

"FAILURE WILL NOT OVERCOME ME, SO LONG AS MY WILL TO SUCCEED IS STRONGER"

"ABILITY IS WHAT YOU'RE CAPABLE OF DOING. MOTIVATION DETERMINES WHAT YOU DO. ATTITUDE DETERMINES HOW WELL YOU DO IT."

DAY 41

"GO TO THE BATTLEFIELD FIRMLY CONFIDENT OF VICTORY AND YOU WILL COME HOME WITH NO WOUNDS WHATSOEVER."

-UESUGI KENSHIN

DAY 42

"YOU ARE YOUR ONLY LIMIT."

DAY 43

"DEATH IS NOTHING, BUT TO LIVE DEFEATED AND INGLORIOUS IS TO DIE DAILY."

-NAPOLEON BONAPARTE

DAY 44

"YOU CAN NOT EXERCISE YOUR WAY OUT OF A BAD DIET."

"SUCCESS IS NEVER OWNED, IT'S RENTED..AND THE RENT IS DUE EVERY DAY."

"I AM STRONG
BECAUSE I HAVE
BEEN WEAK. I AM
FEARLESS BECAUSE
I HAVE BEEN
AFRAID. I AM WISE
BECAUSE I HAVE
BEEN FOOLISH."

DAY 47

"FEAR NO WORKOUT. DESTROY EVERY SET. FEEL EVERY REP."

DAY 48

"STRIVE FOR PROGRESS NOT PERFECTION."

"LONG TERM CONSISTENCY TRUMPS SHORT TERM INTENSITY."

-BRUCE LEE

"WHENEVER YOU FIND YOURSELF DOUBTING HOW FAR YOU CAN GO, REMEMBER HOW FAR YOU'VE COME."

"FORGET FAILURE. FORGET MISTAKES. FORGET EVERYTHING. EXCEPT WHAT YOU'RE GOING TO DO NOW. AND DO IT.

-LOU FERRIGNO

"PAIN IS TEMPORARY. IT MAY LAST A MINUTE, OR AN HOUR, OR A DAY, OR A YEAR, BUT EVENTUALLY IT WILL SUBSIDE AND SOMETHING ELSE WILL TAKE ITS PLACE. IF I QUIT, HOWEVER, IT LASTS FOREVER."

-LANCE ARMSTRONG

"YOUR GREATEST FEARS ARE CREATED BY YOUR IMAGINATION. DON'T GIVE IN TO THEM."

-WINSTON CHURCHILL

"GIVE ME A PLACE TO STAND AND I SHALL MOVE THE EARTH!"

-ARCHIMEDES

"SUFFER THE PAIN OF DISCIPLINE OR SUFFER THE PAIN OF REGRET"

DAY 56

"BE GREAT. OR BE NOTHING."

"WORKOUT. EAT WELL. SLEEP WELL. BE PATIENT. YOUR BODY WILL REWARD YOU."

"SUCCESS TRAINS. FAILURE COMPLAINS."

"TAKE CARE OF YOUR BODY. IT'S THE ONLY PLACE YOU HAVE TO LIVE."

–JIM ROHN

DAY 60

"THERE REALLY IS AN ATTITUDE TO WINNING. YOU HAVE TO SEE YOURSELF WINNING BEFORE YOU WIN. AND YOU HAVE TO BE HUNGRY. YOU HAVE TO WANT TO SUCCEED.

-ARNOLD SCHWARZENEGGER

"DIFFICULT ROADS OFTEN LEAD TO BEAUTIFUL DESTINATIONS."

"IF YOU FAIL TO PREPARE, YOU'RE PREPARED TO FAIL."

-MARK SPITZ

"THE FACT THAT YOU ARE NOT WHERE YOU WANT TO BE SHOULD ENOUGH MOTIVATION."

DAY 64

"I HATED EVERY MINUTE OF TRAINING, BUT I SAID...DON'T QUIT, SUFFER NOW AND LIVE THE REST OF YOUR LIFE AS A CHAMPION."

-MUHAMMAD ALI

"GOOD THINGS COME TO THOSE WHO SWEAT."

"THE ONLY TIME YOU SHOULD EVER LOOK BACK IS TO SEE HOW FAR YOU'VE COME."

DAY 67

"BE SOMEONE'S MOTIVATION."

"HERE IS COURAGE, MANKIND'S FINEST POSSESSION. HERE IS THE NOBLEST PRIZE THAT A YOUNG MAN CAN ENDEAVOR TO OBTAIN."

-TYRTAEUS OF SPARTA

"IF YOU CAN'T STOP THINKING ABOUT IT, DON'T STOP WORKING FOR IT."

"A CHAMPION IS AFRAID OF LOSING. EVERYONE ELSE IS AFRAID OF WINNING."

-BILLIE JEAN KING

"THE ONLY BAD WORKOUT, IS THE ONE YOU DIDN'T DO."

"AMBITION IS THE FIRST STEP TO SUCCESS. THE SECOND IS TO TAKE ACTION."

"FITNESS IS NOT ABOUT BEING BETTER THAN EVERYONE ELSE, IT IS ABOUT BEING BETTER THAN YOU USED TO BE."

DAY 74

"DON'T MISTAKE MOTION FOR ACTION."

"IT ALWAYS SEEMS IMPOSSIBLE UNTIL IT'S DONE."

-NELSON MANDELA

DAY 76

"HARD WORK BEATS TALENT WHEN TALENT DOESN'T WORK HARD."

-TIM NOTKE

DAY 77

"LIFT IT LIKE YOU STOLE IT."

"MAKE TIME FOR IT. JUST GET IT DONE. NOBODY EVER GOT STRONG OR IN SHAPE BY THINKING ABOUT IT. THEY DID IT."

"MAKE GOOD ON THE PROMISES YOU'VE MADE TO YOURSELF."

"THE BEST EXCUSE TO NOT GO TO THE GYM IS THAT YOU JUST GOT BACK."

"YOU DREAM. YOU PLAN. YOU REACH. THERE WILL BE OBSTACLES. THERE WILL BE DOUBTERS. THERE WILL BE MISTAKES. BUT WITH HARD WORK, WITH BELIEF, WITH

CONFIDENCE AND
TRUST IN
YOURSELF AND
THOSE AROUND
YOU, THERE ARE
NO LIMITS."

-MICHAEL PHELPS

"THE WOLF ON TOP THE HILL IS NEVER AS HUNGRY AS THE WOLF CLIMBING UP THE HILL"

"TOUGH TIMES DON'T LAST, TOUGH PEOPLE DO."

"WORK HARD IN SILENCE. LET YOUR SUCCESS BE THE NOISE."

"WAKE UP STRONGER THAN YOU WERE YESTERDAY. FACE YOUR FEARS AND WIPE YOUR TEARS."

DAY 86

"FORTUNE FAVORS THE BOLD."

-ROMAN PROVERB

"NO MAN HAS THE RIGHT
TO BE AN AMATEUR IN
THE MATTER OF
PHYSICAL TRAINING. IT
IS A SHAME FOR A MAN
TO GROW OLD WITHOUT
SEEING THE BEAUTY
AND STRENGTH OF
WHICH HIS BODY IS
CAPABLE."

-SOCRATES

"RISKS MUST BE TAKEN BECAUSE THE GREATEST HAZARD IN LIFE IT TO RISK NOTHING"

-Leo Buscaglia

DAY 89

"PERSEVERANCE, SECRET OF ALL TRIUMPHS"

-Victor Hugo

"NOTHING HAPPENS TO ANY MAN WHICH HE IS NOT FORMED BY NATURE TO BEAR."

-MARCUS AURELIUS

DAY 91

"GOOD PAIN IS CHANGE."

DAY 92

"EXCUSES ARE FOR THOSE WHO NEED THEM."

"EVERYBODY WANNA BE A BODYBUILDER, BUT DON'T NOBODY WANNA LIFT NO HEAVY ASS WEIGHTS!"

-RONNIE COLEMAN

"YOU WILL NEVER COME UP AGAINST A GREATER ADVERSARY THAN YOUR OWN POTENTIAL"

"CHANGE DOESN'T COME IN NICKELS AND DIMES. IT COMES IN DEDICATION AND SWEAT."

-TONI SORENSON

DAY 96

"IT WON'T BE EASY, BUT IT WILL BE WORTH IT."

DAY 97

"EXCUSES DON'T BURN CALORIES."

"THE ROAD TO SUCCESS RUNS UPHILL."

-WILLIE DAVIS

"WHATEVER YOUR 100% LOOKS LIKE, GIVE IT."

"IT'S NOT THE WORK THAT'S HARD, IT'S THE DISCIPLINE."

-ANONYMOUS

DAY 101

"TODAY'S ACTIONS ARE TOMORROW'S RESULTS."

"YOU SHALL GAIN, BUT YOU SHALL PAY WITH BLOOD, SWEAT, AND VOMIT."

-PAVEL TSATSOULINE

"DON'T GIVE UP, GREAT THINGS TAKE TIME."

DAY 104

"NOTHING WILL WORK, UNLESS YOU DO."

-MAYA ANGELOU

DAY 105

THE IRON NEVER LIES TO YOU. YOU
CAN WALK OUTSIDE AND LISTEN TO
ALL KINDS OF TALK, GET TOLD THAT
YOU'RE A GOD OR A TOTAL BASTARD.
THE IRON WILL ALWAYS KICK YOU
THE REAL DEAL. THE IRON IS THE
GREAT REFERENCE POINT, THE ALL-
KNOWING PERSPECTIVE GIVER.
ALWAYS THERE LIKE A BEACON IN
THE PITCH BLACK. I HAVE FOUND THE
IRON TO BE MY GREATEST FRIEND. IT
NEVER FREAKS OUT ON ME, NEVER
RUNS. FRIENDS MAY COME AND GO.
BUT TWO HUNDRED POUNDS IS
ALWAYS TWO HUNDRED POUNDS.

-HENRY ROLLINS

"COURAGE, ABOVE ALL THINGS, IS THE FIRST QUALITY OF A WARRIOR."

-SUN TZU

"DISGRACEFUL, FOR
THE SOUL TO GIVE
UP WHEN THE BODY
IS STILL GOING
STRONG."

-MARCUS AURELIUS

"BREAK YOUR OWN RECORDS."

"KNOWING IS NOT ENOUGH, WE MUST APPLY. WILLING IS NOT ENOUGH, WE MUST DO."

"THE MORE DIFFICULT THE VICTORY, THE GREATER THE HAPPINESS IN WINNING."

-PELE

DAY 111

"I ALREADY KNOW WHAT GIVING UP FEELS LIKE. I WANT TO SEE WHAT HAPPENS WHEN I DON'T"

-NEILA REY

DAY 112

"DON'T TRAIN BECAUSE YOU HATE YOUR BODY, TRAIN BECAUSE YOU LOVE YOUR BODY."

"NOBODY WHO EVER GAVE THEIR BEST REGRETTED IT."

-GEORGE HALAS

DAY 114

"FEAR REGRET MORE THAN FAILURE."

"GREAT WORKS ARE PERFORMED NOT BY STRENGTH BUT BY PERSEVERANCE."

-SAMUEL JOHNSON

"WELL DONE IS BETTER THAN WELL SAID."

-BENJAMIN FRANKLIN

DAY 117

"EAT CLEAN, STAY LEAN."

DAY 118

"THE ROAD TO PERSEVERANCE LIES BY DOUBT."

-FRANCIS QUARLES

"GET YOUR REST.
MUSCLES ARE TORN
IN THE GYM. FED IN
THE KITCHEN.
BUILT IN THE BED."

DAY 120

"EXERCISE IS THE MOST POTENT AND UNDERUTILIZED ANTIDEPRESSANT, AND IT'S FREE!"

"IT'S HARD TO BEAT A PERSON WHO NEVER GIVES UP."

-BABE RUTH

DAY 122

"NO PAIN. NO GAIN. SHUT UP AND TRAIN."

DAY 123

"WHY CHOOSE FAILURE WHEN SUCCESS IS AN OPTION?"

DAY 124

"MEN ARE NOT BORN THEY ARE CREATED. POVERTY, DIFFICULTY, HEARTACHE, OPPRESSION, PAIN- THESE ARE THE THINGS THAT MAKE MEN OUT OF BOYS"

"NO GOAL WAS EVER MET WITHOUT A LITTLE SWEAT."

"THE GREATEST GLORY IN LIVING LIES NOT IN NEVER FAILING, BUT IN RISING EVERYTIME WE FALL.

-NELSON MANDELA

"IF YOUR GOALS DON'T SCARE YOU THEY AREN'T BIG ENOUGH."

-TOM HOLLAND

"YOUR HEALTH ACCOUNT, YOUR BANK ACCOUNT, THEY'RE THE SAME THING. THE MORE YOU PUT IN, THE MORE YOU CAN TAKE OUT. EXERCISE IS KING AND NUTRITION IS QUEEN. TOGETHER YOU HAVE A KINGDOM."

-JACK LALANNE

YOUR GREATEST
FEARS ARE
CREATED BY YOUR
IMAGINATION.
DON'T GIVE IN TO
THEM."

-WINSTON CHURCHILL

"I WILL EITHER FIND A WAY, OR MAKE ONE"

-HANNIBAL BARCA

"STRENGTH DOES NOT COME FROM PHYSICAL CAPACITY. IT COMES FROM AN INDOMITABLE WILL"

-MOHANDAS GANDHI

"THE GODS ENVY US. THEY ENVY US BECAUSE WE ARE MORTAL, BECAUSE ANY MOMENT MAY BE OUR LAST. EVERYTHING IS MORE BEAUTIFUL BECAUSE WE'RE DOOMED. YOU WILL NEVER BE LOVELIER THAN YOU ARE NOW. WE WILL NEVER BE HERE AGAIN."

-HOMER

DAY 133

"STAY DEDICATED, IT DOESN'T HAPPEN OVERNIGHT."

"SOME PEOPLE WANT IT TO HAPPEN. SOME PEOPLE WISH IT TO HAPPEN. SOME PEOPLE MAKE IT HAPPEN."

DAY 135

"DO SOMETHING TODAY THAT YOUR FUTURE SELF WILL THANK YOU FOR."

DAY 136

"WE DO NOT STOP EXERCISING BECAUSE WE GROW OLD – WE GROW OLD BECAUSE WE STOP EXERCISING."

-Dr. Kenneth Cooper

DAY 137

"THE MORE YOU SWEAT IN PRACTICE, THE LESS YOU BLEED IN BATTLE."

"ALL GLORY COMES FROM DARING TO BEGIN."

-EUGENE F. WARE

DAY 139

"THE DIFFERENCE BETWEEN SOMEONE WHO IS IN SHAPE, AND SOMEONE WHO IS NOT IN SHAPE, IS THE INDIVIDUAL WHO IS IN SHAPE WORKS OUT EVEN WHEN THEY DO NOT WANT TO."

"LOOK IN THE MIRROR, THAT'S YOUR COMPETITION."

DAY 141

"YOU'VE NEVER LIVED THIS THIS DAY BEFORE. AND YOU NEVER WILL AGAIN. MAKE THE MOST OF IT."

EVERYTHING YOU'VE EVER WANTED IS ON THE OTHER SIDE OF FEAR.

-GEORGE ADDAIR

DAY 143

"THIS MONTH'S DIET IS NEXT MONTH'S BODY."

DAY 144

"I FIND THAT, THE HARDER I WORK, THE MORE LUCK I SEEM TO FIND!"

-THOMAS JEFFERSON

"IF YOU'RE GOING THROUGH HELL, KEEP GOING."

-WINSTON CHURCHILL

"MAY WE EVER CHOOSE THE HARDER RIGHT, INSTEAD OF THE EARLIER WRONG."

-THOMAS S. MONSON

DAY 147

"IF IT DOESN'T CHALLENGE YOU, IT DOESN'T CHANGE YOU."

"TRAIN LIKE A BEAST. EAT LIKE A HORSE. SLEEP LIKE A BABY."

"BRAVERY IS
WAKING EVERY
MORNING TO FIGHT
THE DEMONS THAT
LEFT YOU SO TIRED
THE NIGHT
BEFORE."

"DO NOT ERASE THE HARD WORK YOU DID IN THE GYM THIS WEEK, WITH WHAT YOU EAT THIS WEEKEND."

DAY 151

"DON'T WAIT FOR OPPORTUNITY. CREATE IT."

"THERE IS NOTHING IMPOSSIBLE TO HIM WHO WILL TRY."

-Alexander the Great

"CAN A MAN BE BRAVE IF HE IS AFRAID? THAT IS THE ONLY TIME HE CAN BE BRAVE."

DAY 154

"THE BEST PROJECT YOU'LL EVER WORK ON IS YOU."

"THE BEST REVENGE IS MASSIVE SUCCESS."

-FRANK SINATRA

DAY 156

"IMPRESS YOURSELF."

DAY 157

"WE ARE WHAT WE REPEATEDLY DO. EXCELLENCE THEN, IS NOT AN ACT, BUT A HABIT"

-Aristotle

DAY 158

"TAKE EVERY CHANCE. DROP EVERY FEAR."

DAY 159

"FALL IN LOVE WITH TAKING CARE OF YOURSELF. MIND. BODY. SPIRIT."

"YOU'RE GOING TO HAVE
TO LET IT HURT. LET IT
SUCK. THE HARDER YOU
WORK, THE BETTER YOU
WILL LOOK. YOUR
APPEARANCE ISN'T
PARALLEL TO HOW
HEAVY YOU LIFT, IT'S
PARALLEL TO HOW
HARD YOU WORK."

-JOE MANGANIELLO

"THE HARD PART IS NOT THE EXERCISE OR NUTRITION. THE HARD PART IS YOUR MIND."

"ALL THINGS ARE DIFFICULT BEFORE THEY'RE EASY."

DAY 163

"THE SECRET TO GETTING AHEAD IS GETTING STARTED."

"FIRE IS THE TEST OF GOLD; ADVERSITY, OF STRONG MEN."

-SENECA

"I AM A SLOW WALKER, BUT I NEVER WALK BACK."

-ABRAHAM LINCOLN

"IF YOU'RE TIRED OF STARTING OVER, STOP GIVING UP."

"TODAY IS THE PERFECT DAY TO CORRECT YESTERDAY'S MISTAKES."

DAY 168

"FROM HERE BEGINS THE BATTLE."

"WHEN YOU DIE, YOU WILL COME FACE TO FACE WITH THE MAN YOU COULD HAVE BECOME."

"IT DOES NOT MATTER HOW SLOWLY YOU GO, AS LONG AS YOU DO NOT STOP.

-CONFUCIUS

DAY 171

"THERE COMES A CERTAIN POINT IN LIFE WHEN YOU HAVE TO STOP BLAMING OTHER PEOPLE FOR HOW YOU FEEL OR THE MISFORTUNES IN YOUR LIFE. YOU CAN'T GO THROUGH LIFE OBSESSING ABOUT WHAT MIGHT HAVE BEEN."

-HUGH JACKMAN

"IN THE MIDDLE OF DIFFICULTY LIES OPPORTUNITY."

-ALBERT EINSTEIN

DAY 173

"VICTORY BELONGS TO THE MOST PERSEVERING."

"ONCE YOU CAN CONTROL YOUR MIND, YOU CAN CONTROL YOUR BODY."

DAY 175

"SWEAT IS MAGIC, COVER YOURSELF IN IT DAILY TO GRANT YOUR WISHES."

DAY 176

"WELL BEGUN IS HALF DONE."

DAY 177

"A SMOOTH SEA NEVER MADE A SKILLFUL SAILOR."

DAY 178

"COMMIT TO BE FIT."

DAY 179

"THE BEST WAY TO PREDICT THE FUTURE IS TO CREATE IT.

"SHOW ME A
THOROUGHLY
SATISFIED MAN
AND I WILL SHOW
YOU A FAILURE."

-THOMAS A. EDISON

"FORGET ABOUT FINDING YOURSELF. GO OUT AND CREATE YOURSELF."

"YOUR STRONGEST MUSCLE AND WORST ENEMY IS YOUR MIND. TRAIN IT WELL."

"IT NEVER GETS EASIER. YOU JUST GET STRONGER."

"WE MUST EMBRACE PAIN AND BURN IT AS FUEL FOR OUR JOURNEY"

-KENJI MIYAZAWA

DAY 185

"IT IS BETTER TO LIVE ONE DAY AS A LION, THAN A THOUSAND DAYS AS A LAMB"

-Roman Proverb

"THE WORK GOES ON, THE CAUSE ENDURES, THE HOPE STILL LIVES, AND THE DREAMS SHALL NEVER DIE"

-TED KENNEDY

DAY 187

"THE IRON GODS REWARD ONLY SUFFERING"

DAY 188

"TOO MANY OF US ARE NOT LIVING OUR DREAMS BECAUSE WE ARE LIVING OUR FEARS."

-LES BROWN

DAY 189

"80% OF SUCCESS IS SHOWING UP."

"THERE IS NO SUCH THING AS FAILURE. THERE ARE ONLY RESULTS."

-TONY ROBBINS

DAY 191

"LICK THY WOUNDS AND TRY AGAIN."

"FORGET WHAT HURT YOU, BUT NEVER FORGET WHAT IT TAUGHT YOU."

DAY 193

"MOTIVATION IS WHAT GETS YOU STARTED. HABIT IS WHAT KEEPS YOU GOING."

DAY 194

"REMEMBER THAT GUY THAT GAVE UP? NEITHER DOES ANYBODY ELSE."

THE MOST DIFFICULT THING IS THE DECISION TO ACT, THE REST IS MERELY TENACITY.

-AMELIA EARHART

DAY 196

"TRAIN INSANE OR REMAIN THE SAME."

"THERE IS NO SECRET FORMULA. LIFT HEAVY, TRAIN HARD, AND AIM TO BE THE BEST."

-RONNIE COLEMAN

"PUSH YOURSELF, NO ONE ELSE IS GOING TO DO IT FOR YOU."

DAY 199

"DETERMINATION DETERMINES YOUR DESTINATION."

"SOMETIMES I FEEL LIKE GIVING UP, AND THEN I REMEMBER I HAVE A LOT OF MOTHERFUCKERS TO PROVE WRONG."

"SUCCESS BELONGS ONLY TO THOSE WILLING TO WORK HARDER THAN EVERYONE ELSE."

"UNLESS YOU PUKE, FAINT, OR DIE. YOU KEEP GOING."

"IMPOSSIBLE IS A WORD ONLY TO BE FOUND IN THE DICTIONARY OF FOOLS."

-NAPOLEON BONAPARTE

"GO THE EXTRA MILE. IT'S NEVER CROWDED."

DAY 205

"SUCCESS ISN'T GIVEN, IT'S EARNED."

"A BAD DAY CAN BE MADE BETTER BY GOING TO THE GYM."

DAY 207

"THERE IS NO SUBSTITUTE FOR HARD WORK."

"WHERE THERE IS NO STRUGGLE, THERE IS NO STRENGTH."

"A MAN IS BORN GENTLE AND WEAK. AT DEATH, HE IS HARD AND STIFF. GREEN PLANTS ARE TENDER AND FILLED WITH SAP. AT DEATH, THEY ARE WITHERED AND DRY. THEREFORE, THE STIFF AND UNBENDING IS THE DISCIPLE OF DEATH, AND THE GENTLE AND YIELDING IS THE DISCIPLE OF LIFE."

-LAO TZU

DAY 210

"MAKE THE REST OF YOUR LIFE, THE BEST OF YOUR LIFE."

DAY 211

"SWEAT IS JUST FAT CRYING."

DAY 212

"DON'T LIMIT YOUR CHALLENGES. CHALLENGE YOUR LIMITS."

"IF YOU CAN'T SEE YOURSELF AS A WINNER, YOU CAN'T PERFORM AS A WINNER."

"WISDOM IS ALWAYS AN OVERMATCH FOR STRENGTH."

-PHIL JACKSON

"TO BE A GREAT CHAMPION, YOU MUST BELIEVE YOU ARE THE BEST, IF YOU'RE NOT, PRETEND YOU ARE."

-MUHAMMAD ALI

"NO MATTER HOW SLOW YOU GO, YOU'RE STILL LAPPING EVERYBODY ON THE COUCH."

DAY 217

"GET UP OR GIVE UP."

"MOST PEOPLE GIVE UP RIGHT BEFORE THEIR BIG BREAK COMES. DON'T LET THAT PERSON BE YOU."

-MICHAEL BOYLE

"YOU ONLY LIVE ONCE, BUT IF YOU DO IT RIGHT ONCE IS ENOUGH."

DAY 220

"BE A WARRIOR, NOT A WORRIER."

"WHEN IT STARTS TO HURT, THAT'S WHEN THE SET STARTS."

"ALL SUCCESS COMES FROM THE DECISION TO TRY.

DAY 223

"NOTHING TASTES AS GOOD AS BEING FIT FEELS."

DAY 224

"YOU HAVE THE STRENGTH TO ENDURE IT ALL."

DAY 225

"RISE ABOVE HATE, PAIN, DEPRESSION, THE PAST."

"BODYBUILDING IS AN ART, YOUR BODY IS THE CANVAS, WEIGHTS ARE YOUR BRUSH AND NUTRITION IS YOUR PAINT. WE ALL HAVE THE ABILITY TO TURN A SELF-PORTRAIT INTO A MASTERPIECE.

-KAI GREENE

"YOU DON'T HAVE TO BE GREAT TO START. BUT YOU HAVE TO START TO BE GREAT."

-ZIG ZIGLAR

"ALL THAT ANGER. ALL THAT FEAR. ALL THAT NEGATIVE ENERGY, TAKE IT TO THE GYM AND SPEND IT THERE. THESE THINGS MAKE GREAT FUEL. LET THEM NOURISH YOU AND NOT THE OTHER WAY AROUND."

"YOU CAN FEEL SORE TOMORROW, OR YOU CAN FEEL SORRY TOMORROW. YOU CHOOSE."

"WHAT SEEMS IMPOSSIBLE TODAY, WILL ONE DAY BECOME YOUR WARM-UP."

"COURAGE IS NOT THE ABSENCE OF FEAR, IT IS THE ABILITY TO ACT IN THE PRESENCE OF FEAR."

"THERE IS NO FAILURE EXCEPT IN NO LONGER TRYING."

-ELBERT HUBBARD

DAY 233

"DREAM BIG AND DARE TO FAIL."

-NORMAN VAUGHAN

"PEOPLE WILL STARE. MAKE IT WORTH THEIR WHILE

-HARRY WINSTON

"KNOW THYSELF, KNOW THY ENEMY. A THOUSAND BATTLES, A THOUSAND VICTORIES.

-SUN TZU

"FIRST WE FORM HABITS, THEN THEY FORM US. CONQUER YOUR BAD HABITS OR THEY WILL CONQUER YOU."

-ROB GILBERT

"EVEN THE BRAVEST OF CREATURES HAVE SOME FEARS, BUT IT IS NOT ENOUGH TO STOP THEM FROM MOVING ON THE PATH THEY ARE DESTINED TO WALK UPON."

DAY 238

"GET OUT OF YOUR OWN WAY."

"A RIVER CUTS THROUGH A ROCK, NOT BECAUSE OF ITS STRENGTH, BUT BECAUSE OF ITS PERSISTENCE."

DAY 240

"ALWAYS DO MORE THAN IS REQUIRED OF YOU."

-GEORGE PATTON

"A HERO IS SOMEONE WHO STEPS UP, WHEN EVERYONE ELSE BACKS DOWN."

DAY 242

"EVERYTHING IS BETTER AFTER A WORKOUT."

DAY 243

"A CONSTANT STRUGGLE, A CEASELESS BATTLE TO BRING SUCCESS FROM INHOSPITABLE SURROUNDINGS, IS THE PRICE FOR ALL GREAT ACHIEVEMENTS."

-ORISON SWETT MARDEN

"THROW ME TO THE WOLVES AND I SHALL RETURN LEADING THE PACK."

"IT IS SURMOUNTING DIFFICULTIES THAT MAKES HEROES."

-LOUIS KOSSUTH

"YOU MUST SHOW NO MERCY... NOR HAVE ANY BELIEF WHATSOEVER IN HOW OTHERS JUDGE YOU...FOR YOUR GREATNESS WILL SILENCE THEM ALL."

-UNKNOWN WARRIOR

DAY 247

"WHETHER YOU'RE LOST, BROKEN OR LONELY. THERE IS ALWAYS HOPE, AND ITS SPELLED G.Y.M."

DAY 248

"WHEN NOTHING GOES RIGHT, GO LIFT."

DAY 249

"FALL SEVEN TIMES, STAND UP EIGHT." -JAPANESE PROVERB

"THE RESISTANCE
THAT YOU FIGHT
PHYSICALLY IN THE
GYM AND THE
RESISTANCE THAT YOU
FIGHT IN LIFE CAN
ONLY BUILD A STRONG
CHARACTER."

**-ARNOLD
SCHWARZENEGGER**

"BE BRAVE. TAKE RISKS. NOTHING CAN SUBSTITUTE EXPERIENCE."

"WHERE THERE IS NO STRUGGLE, THERE IS NO STRENGTH."

DAY 253

"BELIEVE AND ACT AS IF IT WERE IMPOSSIBLE TO FAIL."

"IT IS BETTER TO CROSS THE LINE AND SUFFER THE CONSEQUENCES THAN TO JUST STARE AT THAT LINE THE REST OF YOUR LIFE."

DAY 255

"VICTORY OR DEATH"

"PERSEVERANCE IS FAILING 19 TIMES AND SUCCEEDING THE 20TH."

"DO NOT REWARD YOURSELF WITH FOOD. YOU'RE NOT A DOG!"

DAY 258

"YESTERDAY YOU SAID TOMORROW."

DAY 259

"EVERY WORKOUT IS PROGRESS."

"WHEN YOU WALK UP TO OPPORTUNITIES DOOR, DON'T KNOCK. KICK THAT BITCH IN, SMILE AND INTRODUCE YOURSELF."

-DWAYNE JOHNSON

"WHEN SAILING AGAINST THE CURRENT, TO NOT ADVANCE IS TO GO BACK."

-ANCIENT CHINESE SAYING

"IT COMES DOWN TO ONE SIMPLE THING; HOW BAD DO YOU WANT IT?"

DAY 263

"ONE POUND AT A TIME."

"ACTION IS THE FUNDAMENTAL KEY TO ALL SUCCESS."

-PABLO PICASSO

DAY 265

"IF YOU DO WHAT YOU ALWAYS DO, YOU WILL GET WHAT YOU ALWAYS GET.

DAY 266

"THE SECRET TO GETTING AHEAD IS GETTING STARTED."

"TODAY I WILL DO WHAT OTHERS WON'T, SO TOMORROW I CAN DO WHAT OTHERS CAN'T."

DAY 268

"TURN REGRETS INTO RESULTS."

"PUT OFF ONE DAY AND TEN DAYS WILL PASS."

-KOREAN PROVERB

"THE SECRET OF CHANGE IS TO FOCUS ALL YOUR ENERGY, NOT ON FIGHTING THE OLD, BUT ON BUILDING THE NEW."

-SOCRATES

"IF YOU HAVE THE COURAGE TO BEGIN, YOU HAVE TO COURAGE TO FINISH."

"BE THOU ERECT, OR BE MADE ERECT"

-MARCUS AURELIUS

"YOUR BODY IS A GIFT. BE THANKFUL FOR IT AND TREAT IT WELL."

DAY 274

"EVERYTHING YOU NEED IS ALREADY INSIDE YOU. GET STARTED."

DAY 275

"ZOMBIES HATE FAST FOOD."

"THE SUCCESSFUL WARRIOR IS THE AVERAGE MAN, WITH LASER-LIKE FOCUS."

-BRUCE LEE

DAY 277

"A GOAL WITHOUT A PLAN IS JUST A WISH."

"AT FIRST THEY WILL ASK WHY YOU DO IT. LATER THEY'LL ASK HOW YOU DID IT."

"WE MUST APPRECIATE AND NEVER UNDERESTIMATE OUR OWN INNER POWER."

-NOAH GALLOWAY

DAY 280

"TRAIN AS HARD AS YOU HATE."

DAY 281

"YOUR BODY IS A REFLECTION OF WHO YOU ARE."

"THE TWO MOST POWERFUL WARRIORS ARE PATIENCE AND TIME."

-LEO TOLSTOY

"BEING CHALLENGED IN LIFE IS INEVITABLE BEING DEFEATED IS OPTIONAL."

"SUCCESS IS FINAL, FAILURE IS NOT FATAL; IT IS THE COURAGE TO CONTINUE THAT COUNTS."

-WINSTON CHURCHILL

"IF WHAT YOU DID YESTERDAY SEEMS BIG, YOU HAVEN'T DONE ANYTHING TODAY."

-LOU HOLTZ

DAY 286

"IT AIN'T OVER TIL IT'S OVER!"

-YOGI BERRA

DAY 287

"THERE ARE SEVEN DAYS IN THE WEEK, AND SOMEDAY ISN'T ONE OF THEM."

"THE WAY OF A
SUPERIOR MAN IS
THREEFOLD:
VIRTUOUS, HE IS FREE
FROM ANXIETIES;
WISE, HE IS FREE FROM
PERPLEXITIES; BOLD,
HE IS FREE FROM
FEAR."

–CONFUCIUS

"IF YOU CAN SEE IT AND BELIEVE IT, THEN YOU CAN ACHIEVE IT."

-ARNOLD SCHWARZENEGGER

"IT IS BETTER TO STAND AND FIGHT. IF YOU RUN, YOU'LL ONLY DIE TIRED."

-VIKING SAYING

"BE STRONGER THAN YOUR EXCUSES."

"NOTHING WILL WORK UNLESS YOU DO."

-JOHN WOODEN

"HEROISM IS ENDURANCE FOR ONE MOMENT MORE."

-GEORGE F. KENNAN

"BIGGEST LIE EVER; I'LL START TOMORROW."

"TRAIN WITH WARRIORS, BUT FIGHT BATTLE BY YOURSELF."

DAY 296

"DO THE WORK. BE THE PRIZE."

"YOU MAY HAVE TO FIGHT THE SAME BATTLE TWICE TO WIN IT."

-MARGARET THATCHER

"THE GREATEST PLEASURE IN LIFE IS DOING WHAT PEOPLE SAY YOU CAN NOT DO."

"ALL PROGRESS TAKES PLACE OUTSIDE THE COMFORT ZONE."

-MICHAEL JOHN BOBAK

DAY 300

"WE ARE ALL A WORK IN PROGRESS."

DAY 301

"WAKE UP. KICK ASS. REPEAT."

"WINNING ISN'T EVERYTHING, BUT WANTING TO WIN IS."

-VINCE LOMBARDI

DAY 303

"WHAT WOULD YOU ATTEMPT TO DO IF YOU KNEW YOU COULD NOT FAIL?"

"THE HARDER THE BATTLE, THE SWEETER THE VICTORY."

-LES BROWN

"YOU'VE GOT WHAT IT TAKES BUT IT TAKES EVERYTHING YOU'VE GOT."

DAY 306

"OBSESSION IS WHAT THE LAZY CALL DEDICATION."

"WAKE UP WITH DETERMINATION. GO TO BED WITH SATISFACTION."

"RULE YOUR MIND, OR IT WILL RULE YOU."

DAY 309

"THE LONGER I LIVE, THE MORE I AM
CERTAIN THAT THE GREAT
DIFFERENCE BETWEEN MEN, BETWEEN
THE FEEBLE AND THE POWERFUL, THE
GREAT AND INSIGNIFICANT- IS
ENERGY, INVINCIBLE
DETERMINATION. A PURPOSE ONCE
FIXED AND THEN, VICTORY OR
DEATH! THAT QUALITY WILL DO
ANYTHING THAT CAN BE DONE IN
THIS WORLD. NO TALENTS, NO
CIRCUMSTANCES, NO OPPORTUNITIES,
WILL MAKE A TWO LEGGED
CREATURE A MAN WITHOUT IT."

- **Sir Thomas Fowell Buxton**

"VICTORY IS SWEETEST WHEN YOU HAVE KNOWN DEFEAT"

-MALCOLM S. FORBES

"THERE IS NO BETTER WAY TO FIGHT WEAKNESS THAN WITH STRENGTH. ONCE THE MIND AND BODY HAVE BEEN AWAKENED TO THEIR TRUE POTENTIAL, IT IS IMPOSSIBLE TO GO BACK."

-HENRY ROLLINS

"IT IS NEVER TOO LATE TO BE WHAT YOU MIGHT HAVE BEEN"

- GEORGE ELIOT

"NO REST IS WORTH ANYTHING UNLESS THE REST HAS BEEN EARNED."

"WE ALL HAVE GREAT INNER POWER. THE POWER IS SELF FAITH."

-ARNOLD SCHWARZENEGGER

DAY 315

"YOU CAN HAVE RESULTS OR YOU CAN HAVE EXCUSES, BUT YOU CAN'T HAVE BOTH."

"COWARDS NEVER START. THE WEAK NEVER FINISH. WINNERS NEVER QUIT."

DAY 317

"STAY STRONG AND REMAIN UNBROKEN."

DAY 318

"NEVER DREAM ABOUT SUCCESS, WORK TOWARDS IT."

"YOU'RE ONLY ONE WORKOUT AWAY FROM A GOOD MOOD."

DAY 320

"IF DEATH STRIKES BEFORE I PROVE MYSELF, I SWEAR I'LL KILL DEATH."

-CAPT. MANOJ PANDEY

DAY 321

"EVERY DAY IS A CHANCE TO GET BETTER."

DAY 322

"TURN INTIMIDATION INTO INSPIRATION."

"IMPOSSIBLE IS POTENTIAL. IMPOSSIBLE IS TEMPORARY. IMPOSSIBLE IS NOTHING."

-MUHAMMAD ALI

"IF OPPORTUNITY DOESN'T KNOCK, BUILD A DOOR."

-MILTON BERLE

"THERE ARE NO SHORTCUTS TO ANY PLACE WORTH GOING."

"DISCIPLINE, IS JUST CHOOSING BETWEEN WHAT YOU WANT NOW, AND WHAT YOU WANT MOST."

"SUCK IT UP NOW SO YOU WON'T HAVE TO SUCK IT IN LATER."

DAY 328

"ONCE YOU SEE RESULTS, IT BECOMES AN ADDICTION."

"IT'S NOT WHETHER YOU GET KNOCKED DOWN, IT'S WHETHER YOU GET BACK UP."

-VINCE LOMBARDI

"KEEP YOUR HEAD UP, GOD GIVES THE HARDEST BATTLES TO HIS STRONGEST SOLDIERS."

"YOUR BODY CAN STAND UP TO ALMOST ANYTHING, IT'S YOUR MIND YOU HAVE TO CONVINCE."

DAY 332

"CLEAR YOUR MIND OF CAN'T"

DAY 333

"IT'S NOT ABOUT HAVING TIME, IT'S ABOUT MAKING TIME."

DAY 334

"THE WORST THING YOU CAN BE IS THE SAME AS EVERYBODY ELSE."

DAY 335

"THE HARDEST STEP FOR A RUNNER IS THE ONE OUT THE DOOR."

DAY 336

"LET EXERCISE BE YOUR STRESS RELIEVER, NOT FOOD."

"MAY GOD HAVE MERCY UPON MY ENEMIES, BECAUSE I WON'T."

-GEORGE PATTON

"YOU'RE CLOSER THAN YOU WERE YESTERDAY."

DAY 339

"EFFORT WILL RELEASE ITS REWARD ONLY AFTER YOU REFUSE TO QUIT."

"SOME PEOPLE WANT IT TO HAPPEN, SOME WISH IT WOULD HAPPEN, OTHERS MAKE IT HAPPEN."

-MICHAEL JORDAN

"BE STUBBORN ABOUT YOUR GOALS AND FLEXIBLE ABOUT YOUR METHODS."

DAY 342

"LIFE DOESN'T GIVE YOU WHAT YOU WANT, IT GIVES YOU WHAT YOU DESERVE."

DAY 343

"I REGRET THAT WORKOUT"

-NOBODY EVER

"YOU ARE ONLY CONFINED BY THE WALLS YOU BUILD YOURSELF."

"DON'T EXPECT TO SEE A CHANGE UNLESS YOU MAKE ONE."

DAY 346

"WORK UNTIL YOUR IDOLS BECOME YOUR RIVALS."

"YOU'RE NOT HUNGRY, YOU'RE BORED. LEARN THE DIFFERENCE."

DAY 348

"DO OR DO NOT. THERE IS NO TRY."

-YODA

DAY 349

"CONFIDENCE IS THE COMPANION OF SUCCESS."

DAY 350

"WHEN YOU WANT
TO SUCCEED AS
BAD AS YOU WANT
TO BREATHE, THEN
YOU WILL BE
SUCCESSFUL."

-ERIC THOMAS

DAY 351

"CIVILIZE THE MIND, BUT MAKE THE BODY SAVAGE."

"DO WHAT IS RIGHT, NOT WHAT IS EASY."

"WHETHER YOU THINK YOU CAN OR CANNOT, YOU'RE RIGHT."

-HENRY FORD

DAY 354

"FLEX ARMS. STRETCH LEGS. TURN HEADS."

"EVERYTHING IS HARD BEFORE IT IS EASY."

+GOETHE

DAY 356

"WHAT IF YOU FAIL? YOU WILL. THEN, YOU MOVE ON."

"IT'S SIMPLE, IF IT JIGGLES, IT'S FAT."

-ARNOLD SCHWARZENEGGER

DAY 358

"STAND TRUE TO YOUR
CALLING TO BE A MAN.
REAL WOMEN WILL
ALWAYS BE RELIEVED
AND GRATEFUL WHEN
MEN ARE WILLING TO
BE MEN."

–ELISABETH ELLIOT

"YOU MISS 100% OF THE SHOTS YOU DON'T TAKE."

-WAYNE GRETZKY

"WRITE INJURIES IN DUST, BENEFITS IN MARBLE."

-BENJAMIN FRANKLIN

"I DON'T COUNT MY SIT-UPS. I ONLY START COUNTING WHEN IT STARTS HURTING BECAUSE THEY'RE THE ONLY ONES THAT COUNT."

-MUHAMMAD ALI

DAY 362

"TO EVERY MAN UPON THIS
EARTH.

DEATH COMETH SOON OR
LATE.

AND HOW CAN MAN DIE
BETTER

THAN FACING FEARFUL ODDS,

FOR THE ASHES OF HIS
FATHERS,

AND THE TEMPLES OF HIS
GODS?"

"WOULD YOU RATHER BE COVERED IN SWEAT AT THE GYM OR CLOTHES AT THE BEACH?"

DAY 364

"YOU DON'T GET THE ASS YOU WANT BY SITTING ON IT."

"DECIDE THAT YOU WANT IT MORE THAN YOU'RE AFRAID OF IT."

THE END

FINALLY, IF YOU
ENJOYED THIS BOOK,
THEN I'D LIKE TO ASK
YOU FOR A FAVOR,
WOULD YOU BE KIND
ENOUGH TO LEAVE A
REVIEW FOR THIS BOOK
ON AMAZON? IT'D BE
GREATLY APPRECIATED!

Made in the USA
Middletown, DE
07 August 2019